ANGELINA MARIE

Parenting Gen Z and Beyond

Nurturing Resilient Children in the Digital Age with Emotional Intelligence

Contents

1

Introduction

Welcome to "Parenting Gen Z and Beyond." This guide serves as your compass through the complexities of raising children in the 21st century. From digital natives to evolving family dynamics, explore practical strategies, anecdotes, and expert advice that empower you to flourish as a parent. Let's embark on the adventure of nurturing resilient, compassionate, and individuals with a harmonious equilibrium, navigating the contemporary challenges of parenting. Here's to the exciting and rewarding journey of parenting in modern times!

What to Expect

Embark on a comprehensive exploration of modern parenting, with a special focus on supporting Generation Z children. As you delve into this book, anticipate a profound journey through the intricacies of contemporary parenting. From analyzing historical shifts to addressing the challenges of raising kids in the digital age, the book covers a broad spectrum of relevant topics, drawing on valuable lessons from the past and examining the evolving expectations placed on parents in today's dynamic society.

This guide advocates for a compassionate parenting approach, encouraging parents to acknowledge and navigate feelings of frustration while fostering self-kindness. Offering practical advice on active listening—a crucial skill for effective family communication—the book explores the concept of families as cohesive teams, delving into the distinctions between being kind and being nice for a thoughtful reflection on family dynamics.

Presenting a realistic portrayal of parenting, the book emphasizes the inherent imperfections in the journey, dispelling the notion of achieving perfection. It explores love languages and how children express affection uniquely, challenging the conventional idea of parenting as a rigid set of rules. Encouraging parents to prioritize creating enduring memories with their children, this guide serves as a comprehensive resource brimming with practical ideas to transform parenting into a resilient, compassionate, and loving experience within today's dynamic landscape.

2

Who is Gen Z?

Parenting in the 21st century comes with its own set of challenges, and one significant aspect is understanding and navigating the world of Generation Z, commonly known as Gen Z. Born between the mid-1990s and the early 2010s, Gen Z represents the generation that has grown up in the midst of rapid technological advancements, shaping their worldview, values, and interactions.

To better understand Gen Z, it's crucial to acknowledge the impact of technology on how they were raised. Unlike previous generations, Gen Z is characterized by being digital natives – individuals who have grown up surrounded by technology, the internet, and social media from a very young age. Smartphones, social media platforms, and instant access to information have become an integral part of their daily lives, influencing their communication styles, social interactions, and even how they see the world.

One key aspect of Gen Z is their interconnectedness. Social media has not only provided them with a platform for communication but has also shaped their identity and self-expression. As parents, it's essential to recognize that social media plays a significant role in their lives, influencing how they build relationships, express themselves, and seek validation. Understanding the dynamics of online interactions becomes paramount for guiding and supporting Gen Z through their formative years.

Moreover, Gen Z is known for its diversity and inclusivity. Growing up in an era that promotes awareness and acceptance of various cultures, identities, and perspectives, Gen Z tends to be more open-minded and tolerant. This inclusivity is reflected in their preferences, choices, and friendships. As parents, fostering an environment that values diversity and encourages open conversations about different perspectives can contribute to the healthy development of Gen Z individuals.

The educational landscape has also undergone significant changes for Gen Z. With access to vast amounts of information at their fingertips, they have become accustomed to self-directed learning. Traditional educational models may need to adapt to accommodate their preference for interactive, technology-driven learning experiences. Parents can play a vital role in supporting their children's education by encouraging curiosity, critical thinking, and adaptability.

As Gen Z faces a rapidly changing job market, characterized by automation and the gig economy, they exhibit a strong entrepreneurial spirit. They are likely to seek unconventional career paths, value work-life balance, and prioritize purpose-driven work. Parents can nurture this entrepreneurial mindset by encouraging creativity, resilience, and a proactive approach to problem-solving.

The concept of "helicopter parenting" may need to evolve in the context of Gen Z. While providing guidance and support remains crucial, allowing them space for autonomy and decision-making is equally important. Gen Z values independence and values parents who act as mentors rather than micromanagers. Building trust and open communication channels can foster a healthy parent-child relationship during this stage of development.

Mental health is another critical aspect to consider when parenting

Gen Z. The constant connectivity and exposure to online content can contribute to feelings of anxiety, stress, and social comparison. Parents need to be attuned to the emotional well-being of their children, encouraging open discussions about mental health, and providing support when needed. Teaching them coping mechanisms and the importance of balance in their digital lives is essential for their overall well-being.

In conclusion, parenting Gen Z requires a nuanced understanding of the unique challenges and opportunities presented by the digital age. Embracing technology while fostering critical thinking, promoting diversity and inclusivity, and prioritizing mental health are essential aspects of navigating parenthood in the context of Gen Z. By adapting our parenting strategies to align with their characteristics and needs, we can guide Gen Z towards becoming resilient, adaptable, and socially conscious individuals in the ever-evolving landscape of the 21st century.

3

It Seems Harder to be Parent now

Historical impact on Modern Parenting

Throughout history, parenting has undergone significant transformations influenced by societal, economic, and technological changes. Examining the ways in which our parents navigated their parenting journey provides a lens through which we can comprehend the challenges faced by previous generations. The societal norms, economic structures, and available resources during their time all shaped the parenting landscape, offering insights into the unique hurdles they encountered.

Our parents, often the first role models we encounter, can serve as a source of inspiration and wisdom. Their stories, triumphs, and even mistakes can be instructive as we grapple with the complexities of raising children in the present era. Understanding the societal context in which they raised us unveils the nuances of their parenting decisions. Their experiences can be a guide, illuminating paths that proved successful and cautioning against pitfalls that may have arisen.

While acknowledging the differences between then and now, it's crucial to identify timeless principles that remain relevant across generations. Fundamental values such as love, communication, and support are threads that weave through the fabric of effective parenting, standing the test of time. By reflecting on the strengths and weaknesses of our parents' approaches, we can glean valuable insights into refining our own parenting strategies.

One key aspect of learning from history is recognizing the impact of societal shifts on parenting expectations. As societal norms evolve, so do the expectations placed on parents. In the past, certain roles and responsibilities were more clearly defined, providing a sense of structure that, in some cases, alleviated decision-making burdens. Today, the fluidity of roles and expectations requires a level of adaptability and resilience that previous generations may not have experienced to the same extent.

Moreover, economic factors play a pivotal role in shaping parenting challenges. The financial landscape has undergone substantial changes, affecting the dynamics of work-life balance, childcare options, and overall family well-being. Learning from our parents' experiences in navigating economic challenges equips us with valuable insights into managing the intricate balance between career and family.

In this exploration of history, it becomes evident that parenting has always been a dynamic and evolving journey. As we learn from the experiences of our parents and the generations before us, we gain a deeper understanding of the universal aspects of parenting and the unique challenges posed by the present time.

In conclusion, "Why Parenting is Harder Today" invites us to reflect on the lessons embedded in history and the experiences of our parents. By acknowledging the complexities they faced and identifying the timeless principles that transcend generations, we can approach modern parenting with a more informed and resilient perspective. Learning from history becomes a compass, guiding us through the challenges of today and empowering us to forge meaningful connections with the next generation.

Expectation on Parents has changed

The landscape of parenting, once governed by traditional norms and cultural practices, has undergone a transformative evolution. As we explore the reasons behind these changing expectations, it becomes evident that increased knowledge and studies have played a pivotal role in reshaping the standards society places on the parental role.

The advent of the information age has brought forth an unprecedented wealth of knowledge on child development, psychology, and parenting techniques. Research studies, scientific findings, and psychological insights have become readily accessible, empowering parents with information that was previously limited. The democratization of knowledge through books, online resources, and parenting literature has expanded parents' understanding of child rearing and stimulated a collective awareness of the importance of informed parenting.

However, this surge in information comes with its own set of challenges. The abundance of studies and varying expert opinions can create a sense of information overload for parents. Navigating through conflicting advice and determining the most suitable approach for their children can be a daunting task. The increased availability of knowledge has not only elevated expectations but has also introduced a level of scrutiny as parents navigate the delicate balance of implementing evidence-based practices.

Furthermore, the changing expectations on parents are closely tied to evolving societal values and norms. As our understanding of diversity, inclusivity, and individuality expands, so do the expectations placed on parents to nurture children who embrace these principles. The recognition of diverse family structures, gender identities, and cultural backgrounds has prompted a shift towards inclusive parenting practices. Parents are now expected to raise children who are not only academically successful but also socially conscious, empathetic, and culturally aware.

The influence of social media and the interconnectedness of our globalized world have also contributed to the changing landscape of parental expectations. The curated depictions of parenting on social platforms can create unrealistic standards, fostering a culture of comparison and competition among parents. As a result, the expectations on parents have expanded to include not only the tangible aspects of child development but also the intangible realm of creating an idealized family image.

Moreover, the modern understanding of parenting extends beyond the traditional roles of mothers and fathers. The expectations on fathers, in particular, have evolved to include active involvement in childcare and emotional support. This shift challenges traditional gender roles and encourages a more equitable distribution of parenting responsibilities.

In conclusion, the chapter "Expectations on Parents Have Changed" sheds light on the profound impact of knowledge and studies on the evolving standards placed on parents. As society becomes increasingly informed about child development, psychology, and diverse family structures, the expectations on parents have expanded to encompass a broader spectrum of responsibilities. Navigating this complex terrain requires not only a commitment to continuous learning but also a critical evaluation of societal expectations, fostering an environment where parents can thrive in their diverse roles.

4

Its Okay to Admit Frustration

We are Not Perfect

Parenting is a journey filled with joy, love, and growth, but it also comes with its fair share of challenges. The profound truth is that parents, like anyone else, are human and susceptible to moments of frustration. It's crucial to acknowledge that feeling frustrated with oneself as a parent and with one's child is a natural part of the parenting experience.

Parenthood doesn't come with a manual, and each child is unique, presenting their own set of joys and difficulties. Parents often find themselves facing situations that trigger frustration, whether it's struggling to meet their own expectations or grappling with the unpredictability of their child's behavior. The societal pressure to be the perfect parent can intensify these feelings, making it essential to create a space for self-compassion.

Admitting frustration is not a sign of weakness but a testament to the complexities of the parenting journey. It's an opportunity for self-reflection, growth, and understanding. By acknowledging frustration, parents open the door to self-awareness and pave the way for healthier coping mechanisms.

Similarly, feeling frustrated with one's child is a shared experience among parents. Children, in their exploration of the world, can challenge boundaries, test patience, and express their independence. It's vital for parents to recognize that these moments of frustration do not diminish their love for their children. Instead, they provide opportunities for teaching resilience, problem-solving, and emotional regulation—valuable life skills that extend beyond the realm of parenting.

The key lies in fostering open communication within the family, where both parents and children feel comfortable expressing their emotions. Through honest conversations, parents can demonstrate vulnerability, showing their children that it's okay to feel frustrated and that working through challenges together is an integral part of the family dynamic.

In conclusion, "It's Okay to Admit Frustration" encourages parents to embrace the full spectrum of emotions that come with parenting. By acknowledging and normalizing feelings of frustration—whether directed towards oneself or one's child—parents create an environment of understanding, empathy, and growth. In doing so, they contribute to the development of resilient families that navigate challenges with compassion and unity.

They did not come with a manual

A gentle reminder that parenting is a learning curve filled with uncertainties and unique challenges. As parents navigate the complexities of raising children in the digital age, it's essential to practice self-compassion. The truth is, there's no one-size-fits-all manual for parenting, especially when it comes to Generation Z.

Parents often grapple with the pressure to be perfect, to have all the answers, and to seamlessly guide their children through a world that is evolving at an unprecedented pace. However, it's crucial to acknowledge that no one is born with an innate understanding of how to navigate the intricacies of parenting in the 21st century. Each child is unique, and what works for one may not work for another.

Being kind to oneself involves accepting that mistakes will happen, and challenges are inevitable. Parenting is a journey of growth, not perfection. By embracing the imperfections and learning from the experiences, parents can foster a healthier and more resilient family dynamic.

Moreover, acknowledging that your child did not come with a manual opens the door to curiosity, exploration, and shared learning. It encourages open communication between parents and children, fostering an environment where both parties can express themselves freely.

5

The Best Parenting Skill- Active Listening

What is Active Listening?

Active listening transcends mere hearing – it involves a genuine, focused, and empathetic engagement with our children's thoughts, feelings, and perspectives.

In a world saturated with constant information and digital distractions, active listening becomes an antidote to the potential communication gaps between parents and Generation Z. It entails giving undivided attention to our children, putting away devices, and creating a space where they feel heard and valued.

Understanding the unique challenges and experiences of Generation Z requires a proactive effort to tune into their world. Active listening involves not just hearing the words spoken but grasping the emotions and intentions behind them. It's about being present in the moment, asking open-ended questions, and validating their feelings.

In the digital age, where communication often occurs through screens and emojis, the importance of face-to-face active listening cannot be overstated. By engaging in meaningful conversations and expressing genuine interest, parents can bridge generational gaps, build trust, and nurture a strong parent-child connection.

Exploring "Why Parenting is Harder Today" encourages reflection on the lessons within history and our parents' experiences. Recognizing the challenges they navigated and identifying enduring principles that transcend generations equips us with a more informed and resilient perspective for modern parenting. History becomes a guiding compass, helping us navigate today's complexities and empowering us to forge meaningful connections with the next generation.

How can I start?

In the digital age where information flows rapidly, active listening becomes a potent tool for parents to connect with their children on a deeper level. Here are practical steps for parents to initiate and cultivate active listening with their Generation Z kids.

Firstly, carving out dedicated time for one-on-one conversations is paramount. In a world filled with distractions, setting aside moments where both parent and child can engage without interruptions fosters an environment conducive to active listening. Whether it's during a meal, a walk, or simply before bedtime, creating these intentional pockets of time reinforces the importance of their thoughts and feelings.

Demonstrating genuine interest is the cornerstone of active listening. Parents can start by asking open-ended questions that invite their children to share more about their experiences, interests, and emotions. This not only provides insights into the child's world but also communicates a sense of curiosity and acceptance.

Non-verbal cues play a crucial role in active listening. Maintaining eye contact, nodding in acknowledgment, and using affirmative gestures convey that the parent is fully engaged and receptive to what the child is expressing. These cues build trust and create a safe space for open communication.

Reflective listening is a powerful technique to ensure understanding. Parents can paraphrase what the child has shared, expressing empathy and validating their emotions. This not only reinforces that their words are heard but also allows for any potential misunderstandings to be clarified.

Lastly, patience is key. Generation Z kids may not always express themselves in a linear or direct manner. By allowing them the time and space to articulate their thoughts, parents show respect for their individual communication styles and encourage them to share more openly.

In summary, active listening is a dynamic skill that parents can cultivate to strengthen their connection with Generation Z kids. By creating dedicated time, demonstrating genuine interest, using non-verbal cues, practicing reflective listening, and exercising patience, parents can embark on a journey of deeper understanding and meaningful communication in the evolving landscape of parenting."

6

Family Equals Team

Your on the Same Team

The concept and term "A Family is a Team" forms the basis of a harmonious and supportive familial dynamic. In this perspective, each family member is seen as an integral player contributing to the collective success and well-being of the unit. Exploring the principles and benefits of viewing the family as a team, the text outlines practical strategies for fostering a sense of teamwork within the family structure.

Firstly, the analogy of a team emphasizes the importance of collaboration and shared goals. Each family member has a unique role and set of strengths, just like players on a sports team. Recognizing and appreciating these individual contributions creates a sense of unity and mutual reliance within the family.

Establishing open communication channels is crucial for effective teamwork within a family. This involves regular family meetings where everyone has the opportunity to express their thoughts, concerns, and aspirations. Clear communication fosters understanding and ensures that each family member feels heard, reinforcing a sense of belonging.

Defining roles and responsibilities is another key aspect of family teamwork. Just as a sports team has players with specific positions, each family member can contribute in their own way to maintain a functional and organized household. Assigning age-appropriate tasks to children instills a sense of responsibility and teaches the value of teamwork from a young age.

Setting common goals creates a shared purpose that unites the family. Whether it's planning a vacation, managing finances, or tackling a home improvement project, working towards common objectives instills a sense of accomplishment and reinforces the idea that the family achieves more when united.

In times of challenge or crisis, the teamwork mentality becomes a source of strength and support. Encouraging family members to lean on each other during difficult times reinforces the idea that the family unit is a reliable and resilient team capable of overcoming obstacles together.

This encourages us to make a shift in perspective, urging families to embrace the concept of collective effort and shared responsibilities. By fostering a sense of teamwork, families can build stronger bonds, enhance communication, and create a supportive environment where each member feels valued and connected. This approach not only contributes to the well-being of individual family members but also strengthens the foundation of the family unit as a whole.

What role does everyone play?

Navigating the complexities of parenting Generation Z involves recognizing and embracing the concept that a family operates as a team. To effectively contribute to this familial team, it's essential for parents to discern and understand the unique roles they play within the family structure.

Firstly, self-reflection is a key component in identifying individual strengths, preferences, and areas of expertise. Parents can ask themselves what roles feel most natural to them and where their skills align. Whether it's being the organizer, the nurturer, the problem solver, or the motivator, understanding one's inherent tendencies contributes to the overall balance of the family team.

Observing family dynamics and interactions provides valuable insights into the roles that naturally emerge. By paying attention to each family member's strengths and inclinations, parents can identify gaps that need to be filled and areas where additional support may be required. This observational approach fosters an awareness of the family's unique needs and how each member can contribute effectively.

Open communication within the family is instrumental in deciphering roles. Engaging in conversations about expectations, preferences, and concerns allows family members to express their views on the roles they naturally gravitate towards or those they feel passionate about. This dialogue establishes a shared understanding of individual contributions, fostering a collaborative approach to family dynamics.

Flexibility is key in adapting to evolving family roles. As children grow and circumstances change, the roles parents play within the family team may need adjustment. Embracing flexibility enables parents to respond to the dynamic needs of their children and the family unit as a whole.

In conclusion, figuring out what roles parents play in the family team involves a combination of self-reflection, observation, open communication, and adaptability. Recognizing and appreciating each member's unique contributions fosters a balanced and supportive family environment, laying the foundation for effective teamwork in the journey of parenting Generation Z.

What are Everyone's Needs?

Ensuring that everyone's needs within the family are integral to the team's overarching goals is a cornerstone of successful parenting, especially in the context of raising Generation Z. "Family Equals Team" term underscores the importance of inclusivity, recognizing that each family member's needs contribute to the overall well-being and success of the family unit.

Firstly, creating a space for open communication is crucial. Parents should encourage family members to express their desires, aspirations, and concerns. By actively listening to each member, parents gain insights into the individual needs that should be considered when formulating family goals. This open dialogue cultivates a sense of belonging and ensures that everyone feels valued within the family team.

Identifying common values and shared aspirations helps align individual needs with broader family objectives. Whether it's fostering stronger bonds, creating a supportive environment, or achieving specific milestones, understanding the collective desires of the family guides the formulation of inclusive goals that address the needs of every member.

Incorporating flexibility into family goals allows for the accommodation of diverse needs. Generation Z, with its unique characteristics and preferences, often brings a variety of needs to the family dynamic. Parents should be adaptive and willing to adjust goals to meet the evolving requirements of each family member, fostering a sense of equity and consideration.

Encouraging a collaborative approach to goal-setting ensures that every family member actively participates in shaping the team's objectives. This involvement not only empowers each member but also reinforces the idea that their needs contribute significantly to the overall success of the family.

In conclusion, making sure everyone's needs are part of the team goal involves fostering open communication, identifying shared values, incorporating flexibility, and promoting active participation. By recognizing and addressing individual needs within the family framework, parents create a supportive environment where each member thrives, contributing to the harmonious and successful functioning of the family team.

Start your Family Team Wins!

Initiating communication with Generation Z about the concept of family as a team requires an approach that resonates with their unique characteristics and preferences. Here are some tips to effectively start this conversation:

1. **Choose the Right Time and Setting:** Select a time when everyone is relaxed and not preoccupied. Create a comfortable and informal setting, perhaps during a meal or a casual family gathering. This can set a positive tone for open communication.

2. **Use Technology to Your Advantage:** Generation Z is highly accustomed to digital communication. Consider using messaging apps, social media, or even creating a shared family space online where discussions can take place. This aligns with their preferred modes of communication.

3. **Be Open and Approachable:** Start the conversation by expressing your desire to hear their thoughts and feelings. Emphasize that the family is a team, and you value their input in shaping family dynamics. Being approachable encourages them to share their perspectives.

4. **Relate to Their Experiences:** Connect the idea of the family as a team with experiences they can relate to. For example, you might draw parallels between teamwork in sports or collaborative projects they've been a part of, highlighting how each member contributes to the success of the whole.

5. **Share Personal Stories:** Open up about your own experiences of working together as a family. Share stories of challenges you faced and overcame together, emphasizing the strength that comes from supporting one another.

6. **Use Visual Aids:** Generation Z is visually oriented. Consider using visual aids, infographics, or charts to illustrate the concept of family

teamwork. This can make the conversation more engaging and easier to understand.

7. **Ask Open-Ended Questions:** Encourage discussion by asking open-ended questions. Instead of yes/no inquiries, prompt them to share their thoughts, feelings, and ideas about what being a team means to them.

8. **Highlight Benefits:** Emphasize the positive outcomes of a family working as a team. Discuss how it can create a supportive environment, foster understanding, and lead to shared achievements. Help them see the benefits of active participation.

9. **Be Patient and Listen Actively:** Allow them time to express themselves. Practice active listening, showing genuine interest in what they have to say. Avoid interrupting and validate their perspectives.

10. **Encourage Contributions:** Actively seek their input on family decisions. Encouraging them to contribute to family discussions and decision-making reinforces the idea that each member plays a crucial role in the team.

By approaching the conversation with sensitivity to Generation Z's communication preferences and emphasizing the positive aspects of family teamwork, you can create a dialogue that resonates with them and fosters a sense of unity within the family.

7

Being Kind does Not Mean Being Nice

Parenting Generation Z involves navigating a nuanced approach to kindness that goes beyond mere niceness. The following tips and insights can help you explores the importance of instilling values that encompass both kindness and accountability in the upbringing of Generation Z:

1. **Differentiating Kindness and Niceness:** Help Generation Z understand that kindness is a deeper and more enduring virtue than niceness. Niceness may involve avoiding conflict or discomfort, but true kindness extends to actions that promote the well-being of others, even if it involves difficult conversations or setting boundaries.

2. **Teaching Empathy and Understanding:** Foster empathy by encouraging your children to consider the feelings and perspectives of others. Help them understand that holding someone accountable for their actions can be an act of kindness if it promotes growth, learning, and positive change.

3. **Setting Clear Expectations:** Establish clear expectations and boundaries for behavior. Generation Z values transparency and

honesty, so being straightforward about expectations helps them understand the parameters within which kindness and accountability operate.

4. **Modeling Accountability:** Children learn by example. Demonstrate accountability in your own actions and decisions. When parents model accountability, it sends a powerful message that being responsible for one's actions is an integral part of kindness.

5. **Encouraging Open Communication:** Create an environment where open communication is encouraged. Generation Z appreciates honest conversations, so provide a platform for them to express themselves and ask questions. This helps in addressing concerns and reinforcing the importance of accountability.

6. **Highlighting Consequences and Growth:** Emphasize the consequences of actions, both positive and negative. Discussing the impact of behavior on oneself and others helps Generation Z understand the real-world implications of their choices. Frame accountability as a pathway to personal growth.

7. **Balancing Firmness with Understanding:** Strive for a balance between being firm and understanding. While holding them accountable, acknowledge their perspective and feelings. This balance fosters a sense of fairness and encourages a cooperative approach.

8. **Providing Constructive Feedback:** When accountability is required, offer constructive feedback rather than criticism. Focus on the behavior rather than making it a personal attack. This approach helps Generation Z see accountability as an opportunity for improvement.

9. **Encouraging Independence:** Generation Z values autonomy. Encourage them to take responsibility for their actions and decisions. This empowerment contributes to a sense of accountability and fosters self-directed individuals.

10. **Celebrating Acts of Kindness:** Reinforce positive behavior by

celebrating acts of kindness. Acknowledge and appreciate when they demonstrate empathy, consideration, and support for others. Positive reinforcement encourages the continuation of such behavior.

In conclusion, parenting Generation Z calls for a mindful approach to kindness that incorporates accountability. By teaching the importance of holding oneself and others accountable, parents contribute to the development of responsible, compassionate, and socially conscious individuals within the unique context of Generation Z.

Holding the Team Accountable

Holding a Generation Z child accountable for a negative action requires a thoughtful and constructive approach that aligns with their values and communication preferences. Here are some tips to navigate this process effectively:

1. **Open Communication:** Initiate a calm and open conversation. Generation Z values transparency and direct communication. Express your concerns and provide them with an opportunity to share their perspective. Encourage them to express their feelings and thoughts without judgment.

2. **Active Listening:** Actively listen to their side of the story. Generation Z appreciates being heard and understood. Validate their emotions and acknowledge their perspective, even if you may not agree. This creates a space for constructive dialogue.

3. **Focus on Behavior, Not Character:** When discussing the negative action, focus on the specific behavior rather than making it a personal attack. Help them understand that accountability is about addressing actions and finding ways to improve, not questioning their character.

4. **Explain Consequences:** Clearly explain the consequences of the negative action. Generation Z responds well to understanding the real-world implications of their behavior. Discuss how the action may impact others and, if applicable, the consequences they may face.

5. **Encourage Reflection:** Foster a sense of accountability by encouraging them to reflect on their actions. Ask questions that prompt self-reflection, such as "How do you think your actions affected others?" This helps them take responsibility for their behavior.

6. **Collaborative Problem-Solving:** Involve them in finding solutions. Generation Z appreciates being part of the decision-making process. Collaboratively discuss ways to address and rectify the situation, encouraging them to come up with ideas for improvement.

7. **Set Clear Expectations:** Reinforce the family's values and set clear expectations for future behavior. Generation Z responds well to clarity and consistency. Clearly articulate what is expected of them and the consequences of not meeting those expectations.

8. **Use Technology:** Leverage technology to communicate if it aligns with their preferences. Sending a thoughtful message or having a video call can be effective in initiating a conversation about accountability. Use the mode of communication they find comfortable.

9. **Positive Reinforcement:** Balance accountability with positive reinforcement. Acknowledge and celebrate positive behaviors and improvements. Generation Z is motivated by positive feedback, and recognizing their efforts encourages continued positive actions.

10. **Be Supportive:** Offer support and guidance. Generation Z appreciates a supportive approach. Let them know that you are there to help them learn from their mistakes and grow. Emphasize that accountability is a tool for personal development.

Remember that each Generation Z individual is unique, so tailor your approach based on their personality and communication style. The goal is to foster a sense of responsibility and accountability while maintaining a supportive and constructive relationship.

8

It's not Always going to look Great!

Instagram Perfect HAHA!

Parenting Generation Z in the age of social media brings forth the challenge of navigating unrealistic expectations and portrayals of what a "good family" looks like. The pervasive influence of social media can create a distorted lens through which families perceive their own dynamics. It's crucial for parents to recognize and address the potential pitfalls of letting social media dictate their definition of a good family.

The curated and filtered nature of social media often presents an idealized version of family life. Images of perfection, picturesque moments, and seemingly flawless relationships can set unrealistic standards that may not align with the complexities of real-life parenting. Parents may feel pressure to conform to these standards, fostering a sense of inadequacy when their own family experiences don't match the polished narratives depicted online.

It's essential for parents to establish a healthy relationship with social media, recognizing it as a tool for connection and sharing rather than a benchmark for familial success. Encouraging open conversations with Generation Z about the curated nature of online content can help demystify the illusion of perfection. Emphasizing that every family is unique, with its own set of challenges and triumphs, reinforces the idea that authenticity is more valuable than conforming to societal expectations.

Moreover, parents can actively engage with their children on social media, sharing both the highlights and the realities of family life. This transparency helps dismantle the notion that perfection is the norm. Encouraging a critical and discerning approach to online content cultivates resilience in the face of societal pressures.

In conclusion, parenting Generation Z involves navigating the impact of social media on family perceptions. By fostering a realistic and authentic understanding of what a good family looks like, parents can empower their children to value the uniqueness of their own family dynamics and resist the unrealistic standards perpetuated by the online world.

Expectation vs Reality

Determining whether your expectations for your family are appropriate in their development involves a thoughtful and reflective approach. Here are some guidelines to help assess the appropriateness of your expectations:

1. **Consider Individual Differences:** Recognize and appreciate the individual differences among family members. Each person, including children, develops at their own pace. Adjust your expectations based on their unique strengths, challenges, and stages of development.

2. **Reflect on Age-Appropriate Expectations:** Evaluate whether your expectations align with the age and developmental stage of each family member. What is appropriate for a teenager may not be suitable for a younger child. Adjust expectations to match the cognitive, emotional, and social capabilities of each family member.

3. **Prioritize Realistic Goals:** Set realistic and achievable goals for your family. Assess whether your expectations are practical and attainable within the current family context. Unrealistic expectations can lead to frustration and disappointment.

4. **Consider Cultural and Contextual Factors:** Take into account cultural and contextual factors that influence your family dynamics. Cultural expectations, societal norms, and external influences can shape family behaviors. Ensure that your expectations align with your family's values and cultural background.

5. **Assess Communication Patterns:** Evaluate how effectively you communicate your expectations to your family members. Clear and open communication helps ensure that everyone understands the expectations and has the opportunity to express their thoughts and concerns.

6. **Encourage Individual Growth:** Support individual growth and development within the family. Allow each family member to pursue their interests, develop their talents, and explore their identity. Healthy development involves a balance between collective and individual goals.

7. **Be Flexible and Adaptive:** Acknowledge that family dynamics evolve over time. Be flexible and adaptive in adjusting your expectations to accommodate changes in family structure, needs, and circumstances. Flexibility fosters resilience and a positive family environment.

8. **Seek Feedback:** Foster an environment where family members feel comfortable providing feedback on expectations. Encourage open discussions about whether expectations are perceived as reasonable and fair. Constructive feedback can inform adjustments.

9. **Evaluate Emotional Well-Being:** Consider the emotional well-being of each family member. Assess whether your expectations contribute to a positive and supportive emotional environment.

Emotional health is a key component of overall family development.

10. **Regularly Reassess and Adjust:** Periodically reassess your expectations and be willing to make adjustments. As family members grow and circumstances change, revisit your expectations to ensure they remain appropriate for the evolving dynamics of your family.

By adopting a reflective and adaptive mindset, you can assess whether your expectations align with the developmental needs of your family. Open communication, flexibility, and a genuine understanding of individual differences contribute to creating a healthy and supportive family environment.

Staying Still

In times of doubt and uncertainty, the practice of staying still and embracing mindfulness emerges as a powerful tool for inner calm and clarity. When the waves of uncertainty threaten to overwhelm, taking a deliberate pause allows for a profound connection with the present moment. Sit in stillness, focus on your breath, and engage in mindful observation of your thoughts and sensations. This intentional presence helps quiet the noise of doubt, fostering a sense of inner peace and resilience. Mindfulness empowers you to acknowledge the uncertainty without being consumed by it, offering a space for thoughtful reflection and a pathway to informed decision-making. Amidst life's complexities, the practice of staying still and cultivating mindfulness becomes a sanctuary, providing the mental clarity needed to navigate challenges with a grounded and centered spirit.

9

They Love You, I Promise!

What is our Love Language?

Parenting Generation Z involves understanding and navigating the unique aspects of their individuality, including their love languages. Figuring out each other's love languages within the family context can strengthen the parent-child relationship. Here are some tips for discovering and connecting through love languages:

1. **Observe and Listen:** Pay attention to how your Generation Z child expresses affection and what gestures make them feel loved. Listen to their preferences and take note of the actions or words that resonate with them.

2. **Have Open Conversations:** Initiate open and honest conversations about love languages. Discuss how different family members prefer to give and receive love. Encourage your child to share their own preferences, fostering a deeper understanding.

3. **Take the Love Languages Quiz Together:** Explore the concept of love languages by taking the online quiz together. This interactive tool can provide insights into each family member's primary love language, whether it's words of affirmation, acts of service,

receiving gifts, quality time, or physical touch.

4. **Experiment with Different Expressions:** Experiment with different ways of expressing love to see what resonates with your Generation Z child. Try offering words of encouragement, spending quality time together, performing acts of service, giving thoughtful gifts, or incorporating physical touch into your interactions.

5. **Respect Individual Differences:** Recognize that each family member may have a unique combination of love languages. Respect these individual differences and tailor your expressions of love accordingly. What works for one may not be as effective for another.

6. **Create Love Language Rituals:** Establish rituals or routines that align with each family member's love language. Whether it's a weekly family game night for quality time or writing encouraging notes for words of affirmation, incorporating these rituals reinforces the importance of love languages.

7. **Encourage Self-Expression:** Foster an environment where your Generation Z child feels comfortable expressing their own love language preferences. Encourage them to communicate their needs and preferences openly, creating a space for mutual understanding.

8. **Adapt to Changing Preferences:** Recognize that preferences may evolve over time. Be adaptable and responsive to changes in your child's interests and preferences, ensuring that your expressions of love remain relevant to their evolving needs.

9. **Celebrate Special Occasions Thoughtfully:** Use special occasions such as birthdays or holidays as opportunities to express love in a way that aligns with each family member's love language. Thoughtful and personalized gestures during these times can have a significant impact.

10. **Be Consistent in Expressing Love:** Consistency is key in reinforcing the understanding of love languages. Regularly incorporate expressions of love that resonate with your Generation Z child,

creating a foundation of trust and emotional connection.

By actively exploring and understanding each other's love languages, parents and Generation Z children can build deeper connections and foster a supportive family environment based on mutual understanding and appreciation.

It's never too Late to Parent and Love a Gen Z child

It is never too late to start parenting a Generation Z child. While early childhood is crucial for foundational development, parenting remains an ongoing process that adapts to the changing needs of your child. Here are some considerations:

1. **Adaptability:** Be open to adapting your parenting style to meet the current needs of your Generation Z child. Flexibility and willingness to adjust strategies contribute to effective parenting.
2. **Communication:** Establish open lines of communication. Engage in honest and respectful conversations with your child, fostering an environment where they feel comfortable expressing themselves.
3. **Understanding Technology:** Familiarize yourself with the technology and digital platforms that are integral to Generation Z's lifestyle. This understanding enables you to navigate their world and connect with them on their terms.
4. **Quality Time:** Dedicate quality time to spend with your child. Whether through shared activities, conversations, or family outings, creating meaningful connections fosters a positive parent-child relationship.
5. **Setting Boundaries:** Establish clear and reasonable boundaries. Generation Z values structure and guidelines, and setting appropriate boundaries helps create a sense of security and understanding.
6. **Empathy and Support:** Demonstrate empathy and provide emo-

tional support. Understand the challenges and pressures that Generation Z faces, and be a supportive presence in their lives.

7. **Positive Reinforcement:** Reinforce positive behavior through praise and encouragement. Positive reinforcement motivates your child and strengthens their self-esteem.

8. **Encouraging Independence:** Encourage independence and decision-making. Generation Z values autonomy, and allowing them to make choices within a framework of guidance fosters a sense of responsibility.

9. **Continuous Learning:** Stay informed about the interests, trends, and concerns relevant to Generation Z. Continuous learning about their world helps you relate to their experiences and engage meaningfully.

10. **Seek Professional Guidance:** If needed, seek guidance from parenting resources, support groups, or professionals. Parenting is a continuous learning process, and external support can provide valuable insights and strategies.

Remember that every child is unique, and the key is to build a relationship based on trust, understanding, and open communication. Be patient with yourself and your child as you navigate the journey of parenting together. While the early years are formative, the ongoing investment of time, effort, and love contributes significantly to a positive parent-child relationship.

10

Parenting is a Relationship

Good vs Bad Parents

Shifting away from labeling oneself as a "good" or "bad" parent is a constructive approach that recognizes the complexities of parenting Generation Z. Here are some reasons to consider adopting this mindset:

1. **Parenting is Dynamic:** Parenting is an evolving journey, and the dynamics of the parent-child relationship change over time. Avoiding rigid labels allows room for growth and adaptation to the unique needs of your child at different stages of their development.

2. **Focus on Strategies and Communication:** Instead of categorizing yourself as "good" or "bad," focus on specific parenting strategies and effective communication. Emphasize understanding your child's needs, fostering open dialogue, and adapting your approach based on their individuality.

3. **Recognize Imperfections:** Acknowledge that perfection is an unrealistic standard. Every parent makes mistakes, and understanding this allows for self-compassion and a more realistic perspective on the challenges of parenting.

4. **Encourage Positive Parenting Practices:** Promote positive par-

enting practices that prioritize the emotional well-being and development of your child. Embrace strategies such as active listening, setting reasonable expectations, and providing support.

5. **Emphasize Connection and Understanding:** Focus on building a strong connection with your child and understanding their unique needs, preferences, and challenges. A supportive and empathetic approach contributes more to a healthy parent-child relationship than rigid self-labeling.

6. **Promote a Growth Mindset:** Adopt a growth mindset that sees challenges as opportunities for learning and improvement. Viewing parenting through this lens encourages continuous self-reflection and adaptation.

7. **Avoid Comparison:** Steer clear of comparing yourself to others. Every family is unique, and what works for one may not work for another. Celebrate your family's strengths and find strategies that align with your values and circumstances.

8. **Model Self-Reflection:** Demonstrate the importance of self-reflection to your Generation Z child. By modeling an attitude of continuous learning and growth, you encourage them to approach challenges with a similar mindset.

9. **Embrace the Unpredictability:** Parenting, especially in the context of Generation Z, can be unpredictable. Embrace the uncertainty, recognizing that adaptability and a willingness to learn contribute more to effective parenting than predetermined labels.

10. **Prioritize Your Child's Well-Being:** Ultimately, the well-being and development of your child should be the central focus. Creating a nurturing and supportive environment, fostering open communication, and being attuned to their needs are key aspects of positive parenting.

By reframing your perspective on parenting, you create a more flexible and compassionate approach that aligns with the dynamic nature of the parent-child relationship. Recognize the effort you put into learning, growing, and supporting your child, emphasizing the positive impact of your actions rather than relying on fixed labels.

Memories not Checklists

Creating lasting memories and instilling morals in your child involves a more profound and intentional approach than simply checking off items on a parenting checklist. Here's why focusing on meaningful experiences and values is crucial:

1. **Connection and Emotional Impact:** Making memories involves shared experiences that create lasting emotional connections. These moments become cherished memories for both you and your child, fostering a strong bond that transcends the completion of tasks on a checklist.

2. **Values that Endure:** Instilling morals is a lifelong process that goes beyond checking off a list. It involves consistently modeling and teaching values such as empathy, kindness, and integrity. These enduring principles shape your child's character and guide their decision-making throughout their life.

3. **Quality over Quantity:** Creating meaningful memories and instilling morals is about the quality of your interactions rather than the quantity of tasks completed. It's about being present, engaged, and purposeful in your parenting, ensuring that your child feels valued and understood.

4. **Life Lessons in Real Scenarios:** Moral development often occurs through real-life situations and experiences. Engaging in activities that involve decision-making, problem-solving, and ethical considerations provides your child with valuable life lessons that extend beyond a checklist.

5. **Building a Foundation of Trust:** Meaningful experiences and the imparting of morals contribute to building a foundation of trust between you and your child. Trust is cultivated through authentic connections, shared values, and consistent guidance, creating a positive and secure environment for their growth.

6. **Individualized Parenting:** Every child is unique, and a personalized approach to parenting acknowledges and respects their individuality. Instead of adhering strictly to a checklist, tailor your interactions to meet the specific needs, interests, and personality of your child.

7. **Long-Term Impact:** The impact of meaningful memories and instilled morals extends far into the future. Your child carries these experiences and values with them throughout their life, influencing their relationships, decision-making, and overall well-being.

8. **Adapting to Changing Needs:** Parenting involves adapting to the evolving needs of your child. Focusing on experiences and values allows you to adjust your approach based on their developmental stages, ensuring that your guidance remains relevant and impactful.

9. **Cultivating a Positive Family Culture:** Prioritizing memories and morals contributes to the creation of a positive family culture. This culture, built on shared experiences and shared values, becomes a source of strength and support for your child as they navigate the complexities of life.

10. **Encouraging a Love for Learning:** Meaningful experiences provide opportunities for learning and exploration, fostering a love for discovery and growth. Instilling morals becomes a continuous process of reflection, discussion, and reinforcement, encouraging your child's ongoing moral development.

While parenting checklists can be helpful for practical tasks, the heart of effective parenting lies in the intentional creation of memories and the cultivation of moral values. These elements shape not only your child's childhood but also their character and outlook on life in the long run.

11

Conclusion

Beyond Gen Z: Navigating Parenthood Across Eras

We have embarked on a reflective journey that transcends the specific insights garnered about Generation Z. Parenthood, as illuminated throughout this book, is an ever-evolving learning process that extends beyond the boundaries of any particular generation. The acknowledgment of this perpetual evolution is both a testament to the dynamic nature of parenting and a call to embrace the timeless principles that underpin effective caregiving.

Your engagement with this book signifies a genuine concern for the well-being and development of your child. It reflects a commitment to learning and adapting your parenting approach to the unique needs of your family, rooted in the understanding that what works for one generation may evolve but remains foundational for generations to come.

As we bid farewell to the exploration of parenting within the context of Gen Z, we carry forward a wealth of insights that serve as a compass for navigating the uncharted territories of parenthood. The tips and guidance offered within these pages extend beyond the specifics of any era, forming a reservoir of wisdom that can be drawn upon by parents for generations beyond Gen Z.

In essence, this conclusion invites you to view yourself as part of a continuum of caregivers, contributing to the ongoing narrative of parenthood. The enduring principles of love, understanding, communication, and adaptability are the cornerstones upon which strong, supportive families are built. As you continue your parenting journey, remember that the lessons learned here are not confined to a single chapter or a specific time frame—they resonate across eras, providing a foundation for creating lasting bonds and nurturing the well-being of generations yet to come.

If you found this book helpful we ask that you leave a review in Amazon so that others can find this helpful information. Parents empowering parents!

12

Resources

Nurturing trust and open Communication: A guide to raising Gen Z kids in 2023. (n.d.). Families. https://vocal.media/families/nurturing-trust-and-open-communication-a-guide-to-raising-gen-z-kids-in-2023

TEDx Talks. (2022, May 16). *The difference between Gen-Z and everyone else | Mark Zides | TEDxBabsonCollege* [Video]. YouTube. https://www.youtube.com/watch?v=cmxHUXKS9fM

The world of "Generation Z" children: Some Do's and Don'ts' for Parents. . . – TRANZEND CONSULTING. (n.d.). https://www.tranzendconsulting.com/the-world-of-generation-z-children-some-dos-and-donts-for-parents/

Quenza. (2023, October 4). *Empowering Parents: The Power of Motivational Interviewing - Quenza.* https://quenza.com/blog/knowledge-base/motivational-interviewing-for-parents/

In developing ideas for this book, I utilized ChatGPT, a language model created by OpenAI, for brainstorming and creative input.